No Hogwash Cholesterol

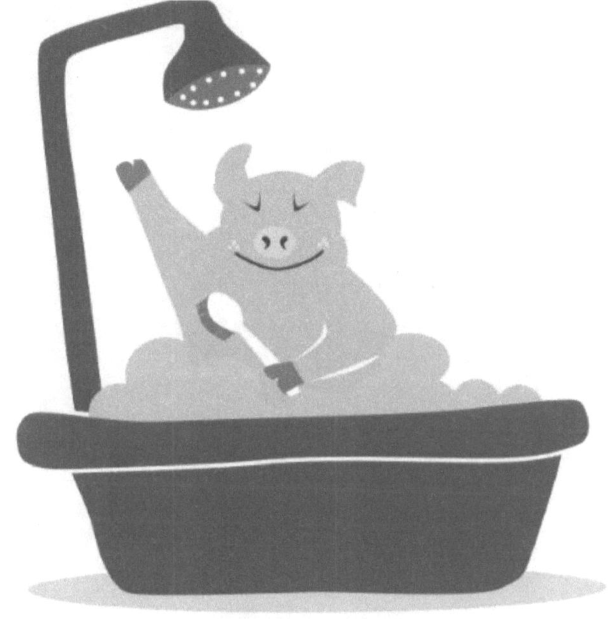

Natural Healing

By: Michael Von Irvin, MBA, BSN, RN

*It is not the strongest of the species that survives, not the most
intelligent that survives. It is the one that is the most adaptable to
change.*
—Charles Darwin

Testimonials
For Michael Von Irvin

Michael
"My pleasure to add a distinguished professional, such as yourself, to my circle of friends. All the best to you and your loved ones."
Father of Steve Job's Founder Of Apple Computers
John Jandali

Author • "America's #1 Marketing Wizard" •
• "The Deal Maker" • "Master Negotiator"
A lot of people are saying great things about Mike Von Irvin.

Former New York City Healthcare executive. Former VP of AlphaCare and Director of Marketing for MLTC Consulting. Serial Entrepreneur.

Past appearances with Geraldo Rivera, Thomas Mesereau (Michael Jackson's Attorney), Tracy Morgan, Prince Royce, Rafael Furcal and many other celebrities, politicians, and sports stars.

BRANDING–My friend marketing whiz Michael Von Irvin says branding is pointless without good Copywriting to back it up. I think he's right.
—David Garfinkel (copywriting legend)

John Fleck
Owner
Wanted to give a shout out to Michael Von Irvin. In one day his coaching and guidance has made a huge difference in the direction of my business.

—Brad Szollose with Michael Von Irvin.

To work with Michael Von Irvin or make comments contact
help@writersprofitguide.com

My second business meeting in the city was with businessman, speaker and trainer Michael Von Irvin and his wife Bella.

Some of our clients have included large healthcare plans such as AlphaCare NY - now Magellan Health. Fitango - innovative patient engagement solutions help to reduce costly readmissions and improve outcomes - NY, Special Touch Homecare LHCSA NY, ASDC, MD's, Nurse Practitioner Groups, FESCO Fire Equipment Company Birmingham/Atlanta/International, Irvin Brother's World Imports, IFPA - International Fire Protection Academy, Hood Master, Southern Fire Solutions, NAFFCO - Dubai, Exit Logic, Jessup Mfg - Chicago, MeridianRx (PBM) - Detroit, and other Healthcare Plans, Providers, Clarity, Tyco, SimplexGrinnell, FireMaster, Clinical, IT, Businesses, Marketing Related Companies, US Military Iraq.

Introduction

This book is not meant to be a masterpiece of grammar. There may be grammatical mistakes. In the spirit of No Hogwash Books, we just try to get straight to the point and to hammer these points home. We are honored that you chose this book to read and study.

REMEMBER: It is what you get out of a book that is important. This book is not meant to cover all portions of the subject. It is meant to help you. In order to learn more and grow more we also have courses designed for each subject of interest.

Thanks so much. We are very grateful to consider you a friend.

For more info visit **www.michaelvonirvin.com**
Or **www.nohogwashbooks.com**

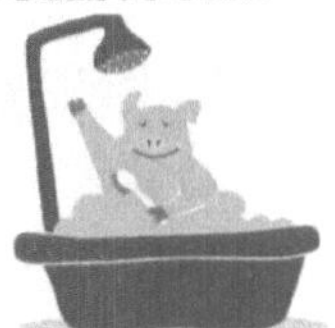

If you are going to make a real change for the better, it will not be easy at first. And know this…..there are a lot of people who are looking out for your best interest. However, there are also a lot of people who will try to control you. I had to break free of negative people and learn how to live my life to the fullest.

-   Michael Von Irvin

Thank you for purchasing this eBook.

To work with Michael Von Irvin or make comments contact
help@writersprofitguide.com

Sign up for my FREE eNewsletter and receive special offers, access to bonus content, and info on the latest new releases and other great eBooks from Michael Von Irvin

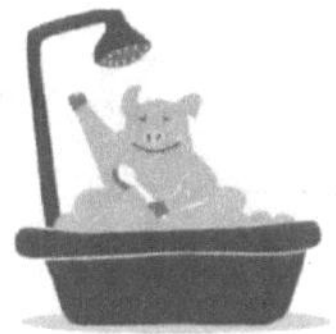

visit us online to sign up

at **www.michaelvonirvin.com**

To work with Michael Von Irvin or make comments contact
help@writersprofitguide.com

No Hogwash Cholesterol

The Healthy Way to Get a Handle on Cholesterol

Michael Von Irvin, MBA, BSN, RN

To work with Michael Von Irvin or make comments contact
help@writersprofitguide.com

Table of Contents

To work with Michael Von Irvin or make comments contact

help@writersprofitguide.com

Disclaimer

Nothing in this book should be construed to be medical advice or even the advice of a nutritionist or dietician. All of the comments herein are from personal experience. The author is absolved from any responsibility regarding any results from those who carry out the suggestions related in this book. Each reader is responsible for his or her own actions.

To work with Michael Von Irvin or make comments contact
help@writersprofitguide.com

Introduction

In England during the 1800s persons ate lots of saturated fats like butter, lard, meat, milk and eggs and there were almost no heart attacks discovered by reviewing London hospital records.

http://www.newswithviews.com/Howenstine/james23.htm

Sobering Statistics

Heart disease in America is extensive and widespread. Most people are trying their level best to do what all the doctors are telling everyone to do and yet the numbers continue to escalate. Here are a few of the sobering and almost frightening statistics:

- About 600,000 people die of heart disease in the United States every year–that's 1 in every 4 deaths.

- Heart disease is the leading cause of death for both men and women. More than half of the deaths due to heart disease in 2009 were in men.

- Coronary heart disease is the most common type of heart disease, killing more than 385,000 people annually.

- Every year about 715,000 Americans have a heart attack. Of these, 525,000 are a first heart attack and

190,000 happen in people who have already had a heart attack.

- Coronary heart disease alone costs the United States $108.9 billion each year. This total includes the cost of health care services, medications, and lost productivity.

http://www.cdc.gov/heartdisease/facts.htm

Hundreds of thousands of deaths, a lower quality of life, lost work opportunities, money spent on doctors, hospitals and medication – these are disturbing numbers by anyone's estimation.

In previous generations higher death rates were caused by infectious diseases. Some of these diseases were passed from person to person. Some, however, were transmitted via bites from insects or animals. Still others were the results consuming contaminated food or water.

The three most prevalent causes of death in the early 1900s were pneumonia/influenza, tuberculosis, and diarrhea/enteritis. Infectious (communicable) diseases were the cause for about 60 percent of deaths. During this same time period, heart disease and cancer were down the list at four and eight respectively as causes of death. These statistics have turned around until today heart disease and cancer top the list.

In 2000, a paper in the *Journal of the American Medical Association* stated that the leading causes of death in the U.S. were directly *related* to:

- Tobacco Use

- Poor Diet

- Physical Inactivity

- Alcohol Abuse

- Infection

- Toxic Agents

- Motor Vehicle Accidents

- Firearms

- Sexual Behaviors

- Illicit Drug Use

The prevalent point here is that many factors on the list above can be altered by making changes in lifestyle. In other words, by taking greater responsibility for our own health and well being.

Billions Spent on Drugs

During this era when the causes of death and disease have been transitioning, the sale of prescription drugs has skyrocketed as the pharmaceutical industry has mushroomed. Money spent in the U.S. on prescriptions and over-the-counter medications is in the billions of dollars.

Because this book is specifically about understanding cholesterol, let's look at the main drug prescribed for "lowering cholesterol" which is called *statins*. Lipitor is an example of a statin.

At the present time statin drugs are the *most widely sold pharmaceutical drugs in history*. The sale of these drugs amounts to around $26 *billion* a year. In 2004, the pharmaceutical company Pfizer announced that their drug *Lipitor* topped $10 billion in annual sales. It was the very first prescription drug to ever do so. These statistics give a clear indication that a large part of our society struggle with heart problems.

What's Wrong With This Picture?

So now we have this picture. We are faced with an ever growing number of diseases that are preventable (or at least controllable) by lifestyle changes; we are faced with an onslaught of promotional advertising claiming that lowering cholesterol prevents heart disease; we have millions of people spending billions of dollars on drugs to make that happen – and all the while the number of people suffering from heart disease continues to grow.

Something is wrong here.

What is it that can correct this out of focus scenario? That's what *The Healthy Way to Understand Cholesterol* is all about.

To work with Michael Von Irvin or make comments contact
help@writersprofitguide.com

Chapter 1
What is Cholesterol?

Cholesterol *Must* Be Lowered

You see it everywhere. Food packages of all sorts and sizes on the store shelves boldly proclaiming: *no cholesterol,* or *low cholesterol.* If all a person ever knew about cholesterol was what they learned from media promotions, the family doctor, pharmaceutical advertisements, and the medical community at large, their conclusion would be that cholesterol is bad. They may not quite be sure why it is bad, but just that it is bad.

Because it is bad, the premise is that in order to be healthy a person's cholesterol numbers *must* be lowered. To achieve those *lower numbers* it nearly always involves a prescription. The main prescription to achieve that goal, as mentioned in the Introduction, is statins.

No one stops to ask if this need for every person to lower their cholesterol is true. Nor do they ask if the drugs are truly necessary. Or if such prescriptions are effectively preventing stroke and heart attacks. Or even if the drugs are completely safe.

What is it about cholesterol that makes it so evil? Let's take a look at the facts.

The Many Functions of Cholesterol

Cholesterol is a waxy, fat-like nutrient that is produced mainly by the liver. Contrary to what is being touted, cholesterol is absolutely necessary for the function of muscles, nerve cells, and the brain. Your body actually manufactures cholesterol which means it has a natural occurrence within the body system. Your body is able to produce all of the healthy cholesterol that is necessary which is about 3,000 milligrams a day. It is also derived from animal products included in your diet.

If we know that the body produces cholesterol naturally, the next question would be *why*? What are the main functions that cholesterol performs? Below is an informative list:

- Cholesterol is produced by almost every cell in the body.

- Cholesterol in cell membranes makes cells waterproof so there can be a different chemistry on the inside and the outside of the cell.

- Cholesterol is nature's repair substance, used to repair wounds, including tears and irritations in the arteries.

- Many important hormones are made of cholesterol, including hormones that regulate mineral metabolism and blood sugar, hormones that help us deal with stress, and all the sex hormones, such as testosterone, estrogen and progesterone.

- Cholesterol is vital to the function of the brain and nervous system.

- Cholesterol protects us against depression; it plays a role in the utilization of seratonin, the body's "feel-good" chemical.

- The bile salts, needed for the digestion of fats, are made from cholesterol.

- Cholesterol is the precursor of vitamin D, which is formed by the action of ultra-violet (UV-B) light on cholesterol in the skin.

- Cholesterol is a powerful antioxidant that protects us against free radicals and therefore against cancer.

- Cholesterol, especially LDL-cholesterol (the so-called bad cholesterol), helps fight infection.

This is a fairly impressive list for something that has been said to be so *bad*. But there's more. As cholesterol circulates in the blood stream it binds to a protein known as *lipoproteins*. *Lipos* simply means *fat* in Greek. LDL refers to low-density lipoprotein cholesterol. HDL is high-density lipoprotein. Low-density is now known as *bad cholesterol*, and high-density is known as *good cholesterol*.

Even though, as mentioned, cholesterol is absolutely essential for the body to function as it was designed to do, still high levels of lipoprotein can become harmful. They can create plaque in the arteries (the vessels through which oxygenated blood reaches all the body's cells) which works to slow down blood flow.

Even more dangerous is what is known as *unstable* plaque which when it ruptures the body tries to wall off the injury by forming a blood clot. If the clot blocks blood flow in the brain, a stroke occurs; if it blocks blood flow in the heart, a heart attack occurs.

Your Body's Cholesterol-Monitoring System

Each person's body is different which means some people will be more sensitive to their diet-attained cholesterol than others. Because our bodies are smart, when you eat large amounts of high-cholesterol foods, the liver takes the cue and subsequently reduces its cholesterol production. This mechanism is designed to keep cholesterol at a healthy level. Problems arise when a person continually, day after day, consumes foods that are high in cholesterol. This makes the liver's cholesterol-monitoring system go a little haywire. In other words, our bodies are created to keep things in order and balance. Due to the lack of knowledge or understanding of what the body needs and how it functions, we frustrate and thwart our monitoring systems. (The monitoring system mentioned here is only one of dozens within the body.)

When the system goes haywire, and cholesterol numbers escalate, we exacerbate the problem by *fixing* it with a prescription. Instead of going to the root of the problem, we apply a band-aid.

Cholesterol's Relationship to Heart Disease

Yet another interesting aspect that you need to know about cholesterol – in spite of all the media attention it receives – it plays a small part in achieving optimum health. While it's true that good cholesterol is important for optimum health, if it is singled out without taking other systems of the body into consideration, everything will soon be out of kilter.

In this chapter, we've clearly established that 1) the human body naturally produces cholesterol, and 2) cholesterol plays a number of important roles in several different organ systems. If this is true – and it is – at what point did cholesterol become such a villain, and why?

Chapter 2
How and When Did Cholesterol Become the Villain?

The big question that has yet to be answered with total certainty is this: is there a clear connection between dietary cholesterol and blood cholesterol?

Yet another question that has never been answered with total certainty: what direct affect (if any) does cholesterol have on heart health or heart disease?

In spite of the fact that there have been no clear answers to these basic questions, still and yet there has been an ongoing torrent of media indoctrination that cholesterol is the biggest and worst cause of heart disease, and one of the best ways to be *safe* from heart disease is to *lower* your cholesterol. When did this thinking arrive on the scene?

The article excerpt below gives a glimpse:

> In 1953, Dr. Ancel Keys published a seminal paper that serves as the basis for nearly all of the initial scientific support for the Cholesterol Theory. The study is known as the Seven Countries Study, that linked the consumption of dietary fat to coronary heart disease. What you may not know is that when Keys published his analysis that claimed to prove the link between dietary fats and coronary heart disease (CHD), he selectively analyzed information from only seven countries to prove his correlation, rather than comparing all the data available at the time -- from 22 countries.

As you might suspect, the studies he excluded were those that did not fit with his hypothesis, namely those that showed a low percentage fat in their diet and a high incidence of death from CHD as well as those with a high-fat diet and low incidence of CHD. If all 22 countries had been analyzed, there would have been no correlation found whatsoever; it should have been called the 22 Countries Study!

The nutrition community of that time completely accepted the hypothesis, and encouraged the public to cut out butter, red meat, animal fats, eggs, dairy and other "artery clogging" fats from their diets -- a radical change at that time that is still very much in force today.

http://articles.mercola.com/sites/articles/archive/2011/10/22/debunking-the-science-behind-lowering-cholesterol-levels.aspx

The Framingham Study

The Framingham Heart Study that began in 1948 is yet another study that was cited as proof of the problem of high cholesterol. Over a long period of time some 6,000 people from the town of Framingham, Mass., filled out questionnaires regarding lifestyle habits and diets. The results were said to identify the risk factors for disease. These risk factors included smoking, high blood pressure, lack of exercise, and high cholesterol.

In a 1992 editorial published in the Archives of Internal Medicine, Dr. William Castelli, a former director of the Framingham Heart study, revealed this statement:

"In Framingham, Mass., the more saturated fat one ate, the more cholesterol one ate, the more calories one ate, the lower the person's serum cholesterol. The opposite of what… Keys et al would predict…We found that the people who ate the most cholesterol, ate the most saturated fat, ate the most calories, weighed the least and were the most physically active."

To learn of other reports that were possibly weighted in favor of making cholesterol the favorite culprit, read the entire article at the link cited.

The mainstream medical establishment has not relented in the past forty years to claim that high cholesterol levels are the main cause for coronary heart disease (CHD). Extensive promotional campaigns have convinced millions that the only remedy is to reduce the levels via drugs and low-fat diets.

If we follow the money trail, it's not difficult to see that such campaigns have netted billions of dollars for drug companies and companies that manufacture low-fat food products. Meanwhile, it has offered little or no benefit to the health of the public. If, as the campaigns claim, cholesterol reduction were effective in preventing CHD, then it would surely lower both fatal and nonfatal CHD.

While the medical world has helped to extend the life of an individual who has already had heart attacks, it has done little to help prevent DHD in the first place. Additionally, the massive push to convince people to take on a low-fat, high carbohydrate diet has been accompanied by a rise in incidents of obesity and diabetes.

Discovering Good Fats

On the other side of the coin, yet another interesting study took place in 1968 when two Danish medical scientists, Jorn Dyerberg and Hans Olaf Bang (now deceased), traveled to Greenland to study the Inuit Eskimos. They knew that these Eskimos ate high-fat diets (60% of their daily calories come from fat) and yet they had one of the lowest incidences of heart disease and diabetes. His findings fascinated him in that other study groups had lower cholesterol than the Inuits, and yet had a higher rate of heart disease. Those findings flew in the face of the newly (at that time) touted findings about the need to lower cholesterol.

In the face of the fats-are-bad-for-you onslaught, he spoke out about the importance of omega-3 fatty acids, but for the most part his words fell on deaf ears. It hasn't been until the last decade or two that the truth about omega-3s has been taken more seriously.

In subsequent years, Dr. Dyerberg has written more studies on the health benefits of seafood than any other researcher. He came to be known as the "father of omega 3s."

When people learn that *scientific studies* are sometimes sponsored and supported by pharmaceutical companies, and that *big pharma* plows millions of dollars into blatant advertising, it gives cause for anger. And rightfully so. However, the important thing to remember is that each one of us can take responsibility for our own health and our own lives. We can arm ourselves with the facts, with good information, and then take action.

In the next chapter we'll take a closer look at the truth about fats and oils and the effect they have on the human body.

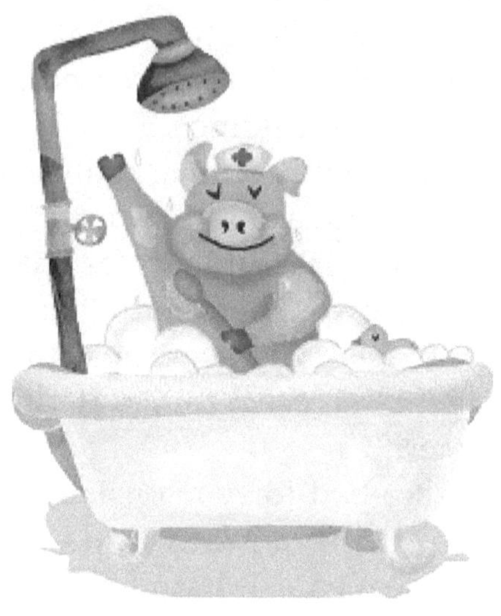

Chapter 3
An Inside Look at Fats and Oils

A History Lesson

Looking back at the studies done by Dr. Dyerberg, one begins to question what fats and oils are all about. It's time for a little history lesson.

The story of the beginning of hydrogenated fats – or trans fats – begins in pre-Civil War days when a candle maker William Proctor, and his brother-in-law, James Gamble a soap maker, joined forces. At this time in Cincinnati, Ohio, home to meat packing plants, soap makers were plentiful. Proctor and Gamble knew they had to be clever to get ahead of their competition.

Because the meat packing monopoly controlled the price of lard and tallow – main ingredients in soap and candles – these two men turned their attention to cottonseed oil as an alternative. They sought for control of the cottonseed oil business, and eventually gained ownership of eight cottonseed mills in Mississippi.

The next step was to create a method whereby the cottonseed oil could resemble tallow and lard to be used in the soap and candle production. Working with a German chemist named E. C. Kayser, P&G developed the science of hydrogenation. By adding hydrogen atoms to the fatty acid chain, this revolutionary industrial process transformed liquid cottonseed oil into a solid that resembled lard. But it was much cheaper than lard.

By the beginning of the 1900s yet another problem faced them. With the emergence of electricity, the demand for candles was diminishing. Now they needed a new market for their hydrogenated cottonseed oil. Since it *looked* like lard, and had the *consistency* of lard, they reasoned why not market it as a food? They named the product *Crisco,* derived from the words *crystallized cottonseed oil*. It was a great idea. One that would prove to be highly profitable.

Crisco Comes to the Marketplace

P&G introduced Crisco to the public in 1911 and coupled it with their ingenious marketing ideas. Their first ad campaign hailed the new *all-vegetable shortening* as "a healthier alternative to cooking with animal fats. . . and more economical than butter." In one simple sentence they diminished their two stiffest competitors – butter and lard.

Next step in their advertising campaign, they wrote, published, and offered for free, a cookbook full of recipes (over *six hundred* in all). And every recipe in it – even the lobster bisque – required the use of Crisco. The idea was sheer genius.

Essentially, at this point, the term *shortening* came to mean Crisco or any similar hydrogenated product and was found in nearly every recipe book from then on. The words butter and lard (especially lard) just seemed to fade away.

Paving the Way

P&G's work then paved the way for hydrogenated oils. Hydrogenated oils became a manufacturer's dream. Here was a substance that acted like cooking oil, when in fact it is only one molecule away from being plastic. The complex chemical process used in the process not only heated the oils to extremely high temperatures, but also introduced several types of metals.

The introduction of hydrogenated oils meant that a wide array of packaged foods could be created containing this substance and they would never spoil.

The lower chance of spoilage meant more profit for

the manufacturers.

Of course at the outset no one, not even the folks at P&G, had any inkling of the health dangers that had just been placed on the grocery shelves and ultimately in every pantry in America. However, in the ensuing years as incidents of cancer, heart disease, immune system dysfunction, sterility, learning disabilities, growth problems and osteoporosis were on the rise, P&G worked behind the scenes to cover up the statistics. It has taken over fifty years to clear the air and to get the truth told.

Dangers of Hydrogenated Fats and Oils

Basically, hydrogenated fats and oils cause a person's blood to be thicker and more viscous. The heart must pump harder to get this thicker blood moving along which then causes high blood pressure. It also slows the blood flow to the brain resulting in various emotional and physical ailments such an Alzheimer's, Parkinson's, ADHD and muddled thinking just to name a few. Tests have shown that this blood-flow slowing effect can occur minutes after consuming such processed foods.

It seems to be more than a little ironic that cholesterol has so quickly and easily been demonized, when it took over fifty years to convince the FDA that hydrogenated fats and oils pose potent dangers to health. Only very recently, the FDA (Food and Drug Administration) declared in its report that there is NO SAFE LEVEL for consumption of trans fats (a.k.a. hydrogenated oils or partially-hydrogenated oils).

As cholesterol began to take the blame for most all of cardiovascular disease and heart problems, how has the medical world fit into this picture? In Chapter 4, we'll find out.

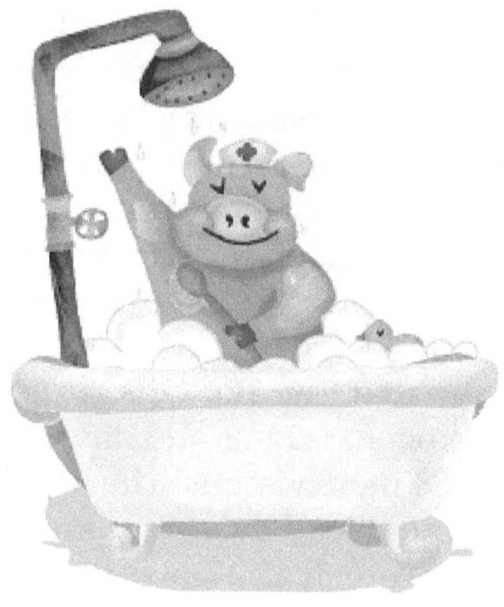

To work with Michael Von Irvin or make comments contact
help@writersprofitguide.com

Chapter 4
Solutions from Pharmaceutical Companies and The Medical Profession

Statins on the Scene

In the Introduction you read this information:

> At the present time statin drugs are the *most widely sold pharmaceutical drugs in history*. The sale of these drugs amounts to around $26 billion a year.

Statins are not *one of the* most widely sold drugs – they are *the* most widely sold. To the tune of twenty-six billion dollars. That is a lot of money. Is anyone asking if it these billion dollars are a wise investment? Are the results worth this investment? And what are statins anyway?

It's a fairly safe bet that when medical scientists come up with a medical problem, the pharmaceutical companies will immediately be on the scene to create a saleable prescription to solve the problem. This has typically been the case in a number of areas. Cholesterol is no exception.

The first statin medications designed specifically to *lower* cholesterol were approved in the U.S. in 1987. Statin drugs work by inhibiting the enzyme *HMG-CoA reductase*. In scientific terms statins are known as HMG-CoA reductase inhibitors. As with many drugs that interfere with natural processes, statins inhibit more than just the production of cholesterol. In fact they inhibit a whole family of intermediary substances – all of which have necessary biochemical functions.

Within a very short time after the introduction of statins, every person who ever watched television, or read a magazine ad, were exposed to the message of fear of the heart-attack-causing *stuff* known as cholesterol. Joining together on the bandwagon were scientists, advertising agencies, the media, the gargantuan pharmaceutical companies and the medical profession. Today officials claim that more than 36 million Americans are *candidates* for statin drug therapy. (Exactly why that would be the case has not been clearly stated.)

The theory that millions are *candidates* for statin prescriptions points to the fact that people are not being treated – symptoms are being treated. It also reveals that no one seems to be searching for the root cause of cardiovascular disease in each individual case. Instead, it is a foregone conclusion that a high level of cholesterol a) leads to heart attacks and b) it must be lowered to ensure good health. Could these conclusions be correct in every case? Why would a person with slightly elevated cholesterol be put on a strong statin drug?

Another fact that seems to go unrecognized and unreported is that more heart attacks occur in men than in women. Add to that the fact that statins work much differently in a man's body than in a woman's. This is yet another clear reason to treat an individual rather than a symptom.

Lazy Consumers

One of the bigger drawbacks to cholesterol-lowering prescriptions is that most people are lazy about taking responsibility for their own health. The thought that a pill will keep their cholesterol *under control,* in their minds gives them license to eat whatever they please. The result is that now there is a double chemical upset to the body – that of the drugs *and* the poor food choices.

What are the Facts?

So what are the facts about this massive push to sell more and more prescriptions of statin drugs? The first fact is that CVD continues to be on the rise in the U.S. We've already learned that heart disease is the leading cause of death for both men and women. That doesn't sound like we are making inroads by using wonder drugs.

In the days when we were fighting infectious diseases, once the underlying facts were discovered, many such diseases were eradicated in a few years. Sometimes less than two years. This seems not to be the case with chronic diseases.

Statins have been relatively successful in reducing heart attacks and deaths from heart disease in individuals who *already have heart disease*. As a *preventative measure* (for which it is often touted) the story is different.

An analysis by Dr. David Newman in 2010 which drew on large meta-analyses of statins found that among those with pre-existing heart disease that took statins for 5 years:

- *96% saw no benefit at all*

- *1.2% (1 in 83) had their lifespan extended (were saved from a fatal heart attack)*

- *2.6% (1 in 39) were helped by preventing a repeat heart attack*

- *0.8% (1 in 125) were helped by preventing a stroke*

- *0.6% (1 in 167) were harmed by developing diabetes*

- *10% (1 in 10) were harmed by muscle damage*

Statins do reduce the risk of cardiovascular events in people without pre-existing heart disease. However, this effect is more modest than most people assume. Dr. Newman also analyzed the effect of statins given to people with no known heart disease for 5 years:

- *98% saw no benefit at all*

- *1.6% (1 in 60) were helped by preventing a heart attack*

- *0.4% (1 in 268) were helped by preventing a stroke*

- *1.5% (1 in 67) were harmed by developing diabetes*

- *10% (1 in 10) were harmed by muscle damage*

http://chriskresser.com/the-diet-heart-myth-statins-dont-save-lives-in-people-without-heart-disease

To work with Michael Von Irvin or make comments contact help@writersprofitguide.com

Taking a closer look at these statistics sixty people would need to be treated for five years to prevent one single heart attack. In order to prevent a single stroke 268 people would have to be treated for 5 years. I've not yet seen this multiplied out in dollars worth of prescriptions, but it would add up to a mind-boggling sum. In the final analysis, would it be worth the cost?

Add to that the chances that one in every 67 patients on statins will develop diabetes as a side effect during this hypothetical five-year period, and one in ten would experience muscle damage. Again would it be worth it?

Side Effects

Here's a list of known side effects caused by taking statin drugs.

- Nausea

- Irritability and short tempers

- Hostility

- Homicidal impulses

- Rapid loss of mental clarity

- Amnesia

- Kidney failure

- Diarrhea

- Muscle aching and weakness

- Tingling or cramping in the legs

- Inability to walk

- Problems sleeping

- Constipation

- Impaired muscle formation

- Erectile dysfunction

- Temperature regulation problems

- Nerve damage

- Mental confusion

- Liver damage and abnormalities

- Neuropathy

- Destruction of CoQ10, a vital nutrient for health

http://www.naturalnews.com/001353.html

To work with Michael Von Irvin or make comments contact
help@writersprofitguide.com

It has taken a few years, but the FDA has now come out with more warnings regarding these well-proven side effects. According to the agency's website, the FDA has issued new labeling guidelines for statin drugs warning users that the medications can cause memory loss, elevated blood sugar levels, and type-2 diabetes, in addition to muscle damage and liver disease.

> *"The reports about memory loss, forgetfulness and confusion span all statin products and all age groups," writes the FDA on its website. And concerning diabetes, the FDA writes that "raised blood sugar levels and the development of Type 2 diabetes have been reported with the use of statins."*

http://www.naturalnews.com/035112_statin_drugs_diabetes_memory_loss.html

The same medication that has been proclaimed as *the answer* for ridding the world of heart disease causes diabetes? How convoluted can things get? Even though the FDA has finally admitted these facts, don't count on hearing it announced on the nightly news. This is why it is up to each one of us to be responsible for this kind of knowledge – and for taking control of our own health.

Testimonies of Devastating Side Effects

Countless sufferers of the side effects of statin drugs have documented their grievances over the years. Many complain of an inability to focus and concentrate, others tell about severe muscle pain.

One fifty-eight year old college professor tells what happened to him upon taking statins. Each morning he experienced pain in his ankles the moment he put his feet on the floor. Barely able to walk up and down stairs, he was losing his ability to actively exercise as he had done for most all his life. But the worst was his loss of concentration. Each new project he undertook as a professor became difficult and then impossible to execute. His short-term memory was so impaired that even teaching the easiest classes was difficult. Depression ensued and he felt disconnected from life. At no time did his doctors mention that the problems might be from the drugs.

At one point, when he was in the deepest despair, he happened to remember that several years earlier a friend of his had made a comment. It was during a dinner conversation that his friend, upon hearing that the professor was now taking statins, said that he should "watch out because statins can do bad things to your muscles."

At that moment of recall, the professor started an online search for side effects of statins and was amazed at what he found. He stopped taking the drugs and was better within a few days. Months later he was again his active self, teaching more classes than ever.

Not Isolated Cases

Such stories have not been isolated cases. The most publicized story is that of Dr. Duane Graveline who authored the book, *Statin Drugs Side Effects and the Misguided War on Cholesterol.* Dr. Graveline had his own nightmare experience with Lipitor and called it the *thief of memory.* Dr. Graveline experienced transient global amnesia (TGA), a disease that involves a lapse in the ability to form memory for a period of minutes or hours, sometimes but not always involving the forgetting of past memories.

His doctors insisted it was not caused by the statin drug, but it was the only drug he was taking at the time. His first experience of memory loss occurred only six weeks after being on the Lipitor.

Dr. Graveline initiated the first in-pouring of patient testimonies of statin-induced memory loss when the syndicated column "People's Pharmacy" published a letter he had sent to them describing his experience. Since then, they have received hundreds of similar testimonies. Thankfully, even though Dr. Graveline twice experienced severe memory loss, there has been no permanent damage. His goal now is to warn others. His main message is that cholesterol is not the villain it's been made out to be; and there are many natural ways in which to keep cholesterol naturally balanced.

Statin Brands

Here is a list of the FDA approved statins:

- Lescol

- Zocor

- Lipitor

- Mevacor

- Pravachol

- Crestor

If your doctor wants to prescribe a statin drug for you, first of all ask pointed questions to learn if such a step is truly necessary. Below are a few suggestions. Remember this is *your* body.

1. If you feel my cholesterol numbers are high, can I first alter my diet to see if the numbers improve?

2. Please explain to me exactly what my numbers mean and how – according to current guidelines – I meet the criteria for taking statins.

3. Please calculate my Framingham risk score and show me what my risk might possibly be for having a cardiac even in the next ten years.

4. If my diet doesn't alter the numbers, is there a safer medication than statins?

5. The dose that you are prescribing to me – is it low, average, or high?

Nothing in this chapter is meant to infer that there is never a need for a prescription of statins. Rather it is to alert readers not to blindly accept a prescription without question. Also to help change the perception that a drug is the quick-fix answer when lifestyle changes can do the same thing – only better – with no side effects.

One of the best ways to take care of your own body and your own health is to understand how the body functions. This doesn't mean re-taking high school biology, but understanding a few basics can equip you to cooperate with your body rather than working against it. As we have seen, the ongoing use of statin drugs often results in an increase of cases of diabetes. How can that be? We'll find out in the next chapter.

Chapter 5
The Connection between Diabetes and Heart Disease

Dangers of Diabetes

In the U.S. diabetes is currently the sixth-leading cause of death. It also leads in being the cause for blindness and amputations. Diabetes can also lead to other health problems such as:

- Heart disease

- Stroke

- Kidney disease

- Kidney failure

- Nerve damage

- Gum disease

Type 1 diabetes occurs most often in children as well as adults under the age of thirty. It's referred to as juvenile onset diabetes. Such a condition occurs when the body produces no insulin. Insulin must then be provided by injections.

Type 2 diabetes is more common. It occurs in adults and is most often no-insulin dependent. This is a metabolic disorder because the pancreas produces some insulin but not enough to allow the sugar to enter the body's cells. At the same time, muscle and tissue cells develop a resistance to the insulin.

Symptoms of Diabetes

The symptoms of diabetes are often ignored; however, the sooner the problem is detected the sooner it can be dealt with and, in many cases, turned around. Here are a few of the known symptoms:

- Urinating often

- Feeling very thirsty

- Feeling very hungry - even though you are

  eating

- Extreme fatigue

- Blurry vision

- Cuts/bruises that are slow to heal

- Tingling, pain, or numbness in the hands/feet

- Irritability

The Role of Insulin

Insulin is an amazing hormone that works almost like a master conductor of a big orchestra – it keeps the entire body in sync. Insulin has been referred to as the "wellness hormone." When insulin levels are too high or too low the whole body goes into a chemical imbalance.

Any form of carbohydrate is eventually broken down by the body into glucose, a simple form of sugar. While the body can use glucose for fuel, if the levels exceed what's needed it become toxic. Glucose that is not immediately used is stored as glycogen in the liver and the muscles.

This process is good but the body has a limit of glycogen receptors. When all these receptors are full (as they almost always are in bodies that are inactive and immobile) other options must come into play. The solution is to store excess glucose as *saturated fat* within the body (i.e. weight gain).

To further complicate matters, in the body of an inactive person who is also a *carboholic,* as soon as the body senses glucose in the bloodstream, the pancreas releases insulin. This released insulin signals the body to store the glucose as glycogen. If the glycogen receptors are full and the body thinks that the cells didn't get the message and releases *even more insulin.*

It's easy to see how body chemicals can all be thrown out of balance. But when a person is unaware of how complex the systems are, they are unprepared to cooperate with the body.

Drug Related Diabetes

> *Hyperinsulinemia: Rise in fasting insulin values by 13 % is seen after statin therapy is started. This is undesirable because high levels of insulin increase the construction of arteriosclerotic plaques over time. Also high insulin values accelerate the rate of development of both diabetes and aging.*
>
> **http://www.newswithviews.com/Howenstine/james23.htm**

The big question for many is whether or not their diabetes is drug-induced. In the statistics provided in Chapter 4, we saw that ongoing intake of statin drugs resulted in diabetes. Why? Where is the connection?

Without going into complex scientific jargon, here is a simplified version. Studies prove that statin drugs can raise the levels of blood sugar in the body. These statin drugs send messages to the liver telling it to STOP making any more cholesterol. This means the liver sends the sugar back out into the bloodstream and now the diagnosis comes back as type 2 diabetes.

The Need to Treat the Whole Person

Everything within the body is amazingly linked together. Again, this is why it is crucial that the whole person be treated by a physician and not just one or two isolated symptoms. This interconnection between statins and the onset of diabetes is a perfect case in point.

Statins are known to deplete vitamin D and reduce the body's ability to create active vitamin D. At the same time statins reduce cholesterol (which is what they are designed to do). The kicker comes when you learn that your body you must have cholesterol in order to make vitamin D. Now you've lost both cholesterol *and* the necessary vitamin D.

CoQ10 The Energy-Maker

Statins also suppress the natural coenzyme Q10, which is responsible for making energy in every cell in your body. CoQ10 is produced primarily in the liver. Most people know that CoQ10 is a powerful antioxidant, but it also has another job – that of maintaining healthy blood glucose levels. (Is the diabetes connection becoming clearer?) When the levels of CoQ10 go down, the body is losing the benefit of blood glucose regulation. (The glucose regulation that was described above.)

> *Additionally, a study published in the American Journal of Clinical Nutrition determined that raising vitamin D serum levels from 25 to 75 nmol/L can improve insulin sensitivity by a whopping 60 percent; even the diabetes drug Metformin® only reduces blood sugar by approximately 13 percent, according to the New England Journal of Medicine.*
>
> http://totalhealthmagazine.com/articles/diabetes/the-link-between-statin-drugs-diabetes-and-cholesterol.html

The connection between statin drugs and the increase in numbers of cases of diagnosed diabetes is no longer simply a theory. Too many studies and too much research have been presented to deny the connection.

It's easy to sit back and blame the system, or the medical world, or the media, or pharmaceutical companies. But blaming will not create optimum health for you. What is it in your lifestyle that is contributing to your health problems? We'll look at a few of these in the next chapter.

To work with Michael Von Irvin or make comments contact help@writersprofitguide.com

Chapter 6
Blame Cholesterol?
Or Take Responsibility?

It's Your Body

At the beginning of this book, *The Healthy Way to Understand Cholesterol,* we saw that cholesterol is not all bad. In fact, the body produces cholesterol because it is vital for good health. Even if you never consumed any cholesterol, you would still have cholesterol in your body. And that's a good thing since it's needed by every one of your cells to produce cell membranes.

It's time for each one of us to do our own research and take responsibility for our own health and well being. Who will ever care more for your body and your health than you? The *politically correct* information regarding the demonizing of cholesterol simply does not hold up under close scrutiny. Take a look at how we as Americans compare to other cultures – cultures that are not overly worried about their cholesterol levels.

People in northern India consume 17 times more animal fat but have an incidence of coronary heart disease seven times lower than people in southern India.15 The Masai and kindred tribes of Africa subsist largely on milk, blood and beef. They are free from coronary heart disease and have excellent blood cholesterol levels.

Eskimos eat liberally of animal fats from fish and marine animals. On their native diet they are free of disease and exceptionally hardy. An extensive study of diet and disease patterns in China found that the region in which the populace consumes large amounts of whole milk had half the rate of heart disease as several districts in which only small amounts of animal products are consumed.

Several Mediterranean societies have low rates of heart disease even though fat-including highly saturated fat from lamb, sausage and goat cheese-comprises up to 70% of their caloric intake. The inhabitants of Crete, for example, are remarkable for their good health and longevity. A study of Puerto Ricans revealed that, although they consume large amounts of animal fat, they have a very low incidence of colon and breast cancer.

A study of the long-lived inhabitants of Soviet Georgia revealed that those who eat the most fatty meat live the longest. In Okinawa, where the average life span for women is 84 years-longer than in Japan-the inhabitants eat generous amounts of pork and seafood and do all their cooking in lard. None of these studies is mentioned by those urging restriction of saturated fats.

The relative good health of the Japanese, who have the longest life span of any nation in the world, is generally attributed to a lowfat diet. Although the Japanese eat few dairy fats, the notion that their diet is low in fat is a myth; rather, it contains moderate amounts of animal fats from eggs, pork, chicken, beef, seafood and organ meats. With their fondness for shellfish and fish broth, eaten on a daily basis, the Japanese probably consume more cholesterol than most Americans.

What they do not consume is a lot of vegetable oil, white flour or processed food (although they do eat white rice). The life span of the Japanese has increased since World War II with an increase in animal fat and protein in the diet. Those who point to Japanese statistics to promote the lowfat diet fail to mention that the Swiss live almost as long on one of the fattiest diets in the world. Tied for third in the longevity stakes are Austria and Greece-both with high-fat diets.

To work with Michael Von Irvin or make comments contact
help@writersprofitguide.com

As a final example, let us consider the French. Anyone who has eaten his way across France has observed that the French diet is just loaded with saturated fats in the form of butter, eggs, cheese, cream, liver, meats and rich patés. Yet the French have a lower rate of coronary heart disease than many other western countries.

http://articles.mercola.com/sites/articles/archive/2002/08/17/saturated-fat1.aspx

These truths are largely overlooked and ignored by the mainstream media and the medical community. But this information is out there for anyone who cares to learn.

Time to Get Honest

Buying into the cholesterol myths places you on a spinning carousel in which you have no control. You become a victim of problematic symptoms which send you running to the doctor where you will receive another prescription. In the meantime what habits control your life that are adding to the health problems that keep increasing?

Look over these listed here and note which one(s) fit your present situation.

- Tobacco use

- Diet of highly processed foods

- High intake of sugary and salty snacks (no nutritional value)

- Drinking your calories – sweet drinks including soda pop (no nutritional value)

- High intake of caffeine

- High amounts of trans fats; low intake of *good fats*

- Lack of fresh fruits and vegetables in the diet

- High levels of ongoing stress

- Little or no aerobic exercise

- Little or no time outdoors in the sunshine and fresh air

- Insufficient sleep

What is Good Health?

It all comes down to whether or not you are ready to get radical about enjoying optimum health. This begs the question, what exactly is good health? Most people have no clue. They believe good health means the absence of a chronic disease such as cancer, or diabetes, or CVD. Yet all the while they are tired, lethargic, running on low energy which has to be propped up every morning with a shot of caffeine. They have trouble sleeping and can't leave the house without a package of antacids in their purse or pocket. Every time they eat their stomach rebels.

Their medicine cabinet is full of prescriptions and their pantry is full of products that are almost totally lacking in the nutrients that are necessary for the body to function even at a minimum of efficiency. Sound familiar?

- When was the last time you jumped out of bed in the morning eager and excited to start the day?

- When was the last time your body was free of aches and pains?

- When was the last time you had a really good night sleep (without sleep aids)?

- When was the last time you felt charged with energy?

If your answer is either "I can't remember…" or "It's been way too long…" it's time to make a few lifestyle changes and find out firsthand what it means to experience optimum health every day. And in the process, your heart will function as it was designed to function. Not because you are taking drugs to lower your cholesterol, but because you know how your heart functions, and what it needs.

In the next chapter we'll touch on a few things that are needed to keep your heart in tip-top condition.

Chapter 7
What the Body Needs for Good Heart-Health
The Inexpensive Way to Heart-Health

Doctor visits are expensive and time consuming. Prescriptions are extremely expensive and, as we have seen, often come loaded with unwanted side effects. But interestingly enough, the things your body actually needs for optimum health are not at all expensive. Let's take a look:

- Real whole fresh food

- Nutrients (vitamins and minerals)

- Light

- Water

- Air

- Sleep

- Movement

- Rhythm

- Love

- Connection

- Meaning

To work with Michael Von Irvin or make comments contact
help@writersprofitguide.com

- Purpose

In glancing over this list what is prevalent in your life? What is missing?

Understand Your Heart

In order to understand the role that cholesterol plays in the health of the body, first we must understand about the heart. After all, it is heart disease that higher levels of cholesterol is blamed for.

Here are a few basic facts about the human heart:

- The heart is one of the most important organs in the human body, continuously pumping blood around the body through blood vessels.

- The heart is located in the chest and is well protected by the rib cage.

- The heart is made up of four chambers, the left atrium, right atrium, left ventricle and right ventricle.

- There are four valves in the human heart; they ensure that blood only goes one way, either in or out.

- Blood that leaves the heart is carried through arteries. The main artery leaving the left ventricle is the aorta while the main artery leaving the right ventricle is the pulmonary artery.

- Blood going toward the heart is carried through veins. Blood coming from the lungs to the left atrium is carried through the pulmonary veins while blood coming from the body to the right atrium is carried through the superior vena cava and inferior vena cava.

- When the heart contracts it makes the chambers smaller and pushes blood into the blood vessels. After the heart relaxes again the chambers get bigger and are filled with blood coming back into the heart.

- Electricity going through your heart makes the muscle cells contract.

- An electrocardiogram (ECG) is a machine with a line moving across a screen that occasionally spikes (or remains flat when a patient is dying). This machine measures the electricity going through a patient's heart. A doctor uses the information to know when a patient is having heart rhythm problems or even a heart attack.

- Heart attacks cause scar tissue to form amongst normal heart tissue; this can lead to further heart problems or even heart failure.

Let's add to this list two other basic factors regarding heart-health.

1. The heart is a muscle. Just as the other muscles in your body need to be moved and exercised, so it is with the heart. The more it is exercised and stronger it becomes.

2. The second factor in heart-health is the need to keep all the passageways clear so the blood can flow easily and without obstructions. This is not a mystery. The knowledge of what keeps the veins and arteries clear has been available for decades. (Hint: it's not through cholesterol-lowering drugs.) Again, the point here is the more you know and understand how your body works, the more equipped you will be to cooperate.

What the Cardiovascular System Needs
Coenzyme Q10

Coenzyme Q10 is a fat-soluble, vitamin-like substance required for normal mitochondrial function (cell energy). CoQ10 has two major functions within the body. First, cells use it to generate energy which allows the body to function. Second, it acts as an anti-oxidant, helping to protect tissues of the body from damage due to toxic molecules known as free radicals. About half of our CoQ10 comes from the fat in our diets; the remainder is produced within the body.

The heart muscle cells have a distinct need for this *cell energy*, hence the need for healthy amounts of CoQ10. Unfortunately statins are responsible for lowering blood levels of CoQ10 as they are closely related to the same chemical pathway as cholesterol. The drug is not selective – it reduces more than just cholesterol. Because this vitamin is so crucial to heart-health, it is often taken as a vitamin supplement to ensure optimum health.

Healthy Fats – Omega-3

In Chapter 3, we learned the disturbing truth about the introduction of fats and oils that are bad for the heart and the entire circulatory system. Then came the low-fat and no-fat diatribe which convinced consumers that all fats are bad for you. This took the subject from one extreme to the other.

The balance comes when you understand about the *good fats* which are called omega-3s. Below is a list of a few of the foods that top the list in being rich in Omega-3 fatty acids:

- Flaxseed oil

- Seeds, flaxseed

- Seeds, chia seeds

- Fish oil, salmon

- Oil, bearded seal

- Fish oil, sardine

- Fish oil, cod liver

- Nuts, walnuts

- Fish, mackerel

- Fish, salmon

Omega-3s have a number of ways in which they support and energize your heart. They work to lower your resting heart rate. This means even when you are under stress, they lower your heart rate a few beats every minute.

Omega-3s also act as an anticoagulant which means the blood will be thinner and keep moving quickly through the system. This keeps the surface of the arterial walls smooth and lessens clotting.

As a fat, it lowers the *bad* cholesterol and yet it protects and raises the HDL or the protective cholesterol. And last but not least omega-3s steady your heartbeat. It remains a mystery how this happens, but extensive studies have shown that sea foods mentioned in the list above steadies the electrical system of the heart.

Healthy Oils

At the mention of cooking oil, most people think of products such as Crisco oils and other *vegetable oils.* However olive oil is the better choice since it is rich in monounsaturated fatty acids (MUFAs). MUFAs are anti-inflammatory and, like the omega-3s mentioned above help to keep the lining of the arteries smooth.

Unlike other oils that are produced from the *seeds* of the plant, olive oil is made from the *flesh* of the olives. Less pressure and lower temperatures are used in processing which preserves the nutritional value. Olive oil is rich in heart-healthy fats and also contains antioxidants. Olive oil is known to be a highly *synergistic* food. This means that when it's added to other foods – especially vegetables – it increases the absorption of nutrients.

Other healthy oils include:

- Flax oil

- Fish oils

- Nut oils

Plant-Based Foods

Plant-based foods are known to keep the arteries soft and smooth. On the other hand animal-based foods keep the arteries stiff and sticky. The incidents of heart attacks following a high-fat meal are so prevalent that cardiologists have come to refer to the problem as the *steakhouse syndrome.*

High amounts of the wrong kinds of fats cause the blood to go into a hyper-sticky state – the vessels narrow, triglycerides in the blood spike, and consequently blood pressure rises. When the bloodstream is bloated with fats the blood-fats peak several hour later and do not begin to recede until almost *eight hours later.* Think of the amount of time that the body must struggle against this unnatural onslaught.

There is no record of incidents of heart attacks directly following a meal of fish, fruits, and vegetables. A meal of salmon, for instance, increases the enzyme that helps clear triglycerides from the bloodstream. We've already seen the heart-healthy benefits of omega-3s. Add to those benefits the benefits of eating fruits and vegetables and you're on your way to fully cooperating with your cardiovascular system.

Fruits and vegetables in their raw state (or close to raw – such as steamed) are full of phytochemicals which is a bioactive non-nutrient. While it has been estimated that more than 5000 phytochemicals exist (many more have not been identified), we know that they are highly effective in the reduction of free radicals in the body.
Many phytonutrients have antioxidant properties that help prevent damage to cells throughout the body. Phytonutrients have been shown to reduce the risk of cancer, heart disease, stroke, Alzheimer's and Parkinson's disease. Eating plenty of phytonutrient-rich foods can help promote healthy aging.

To work with Michael Von Irvin or make comments contact
help@writersprofitguide.com

Additionally, plant-based foods (in their raw state) supply fiber to the system. Fiber is known to be good for the heart, because of its ability to lower cholesterol levels. Also, there is good evidence that it can help normalize blood pressure and reduce inflammation. Fiber also helps to control blood sugar levels, which means anyone concerned about diabetes should up their intake of fruits and vegetables.

Movement

It's a sad state of affairs when the word *exercise* has become a despised, guilt-ridden term. We have evolved into a sedentary society because it's so easy to jump in the car, take the elevator, park close to shopping, slow down in the evening and veg out in front of the television or computer. Not only have we lost the *opportunity* to move, we've forgotten why movement is so crucial to optimum health.

It was mentioned at the first of this chapter that the heart is a muscle. In the inactive, overweight body, the heart is very seldom getting enough exercise. It becomes weak and flabby. With each beat of an unfit heart, a lower volume of blood is pumped through the body than that of a stronger heart. This means the heart has to beat more frequently to ensure adequate circulation – resulting in an overworked heart. Blood pressure increases causing stiffness and hardening of the arteries.

A strong, healthy heart has a healthy stroke volume. The heart rate is slower and a more healthy tone is created in the arterial walls. This is attained by regular exercise. The benefits of exercise are way too numerous to be included in this one book, but here are a few.

Increased physical activity:

- Burns up calories.

- Lowers LDL and triglyceride levels

- Raises good cholesterol

- Reduces feelings of depression and anxiety

- Builds and maintains healthy bones, muscles and joints

Exercise that takes a person into the out of doors has the added benefits of vitamin D (the sunshine vitamin). While there are definite benefits of working out in the climate-controlled local gym, outdoor exercise offers even more benefits. Those who walk, jog, or bike, find more of a psychological benefit from being in the fresh air. Plus the fact that they exercise for longer periods of time than when exercising in the gym. Either way – indoors or out – movement, activity, and exercise could very well save your life. Or at the very least, extend it.

This chapter has made it clear exactly what is necessary to maintain a healthy heart and cardiovascular system. It's neither difficult nor expensive. What it does require is determination and commitment. More about that in the next chapter.

Chapter 8
The Power to Create Health

Take Action

You have been exposed to a great deal of basic information in this book. But none of the information will be of any benefit unless you make a quality decision to put this knowledge into action. Some of the facts may have been things you have already known; others may have been totally new to you, but now you are responsible for what you know.

Many people in this information age are weary of being herded through the medical system with little or no individualized attention given to the whole person. They are weary of the fact that little or no attention is given to uncovering the core causes of whatever health problem might be in question. These are people who are ready to take more responsibility regarding their health and their health care. Where do you stand?

This in no way should be construed to say we no longer need doctors and medicine. It does say we need not be passive when a prescription is placed into our hands.

Prepare the Mind

The decision to make lifestyle changes and to regain your health starts as a paradigm shift. It requires making a quality decision to begin, and then taking a few steps each day, then each week, to make it happen.

By his own admission, Dr. William Sears (author of *Prime-Time Health*) grew up as an *overweight eater* – the *chubby* kid. Even in his adult years his health habits were not good. All along his wife, Martha tried to encourage him to change his eating habits. He refused to listen. But at age fifty-seven a cancer diagnosis caused him to care; hence he began his journey *back to health.* He was now ready to get serious about taking responsibility for his own good health.

Hopefully it will not take a situation that drastic that moves you to action. Perhaps it will simply be because you are sick and tired of being sick and tired.

For many people the idea of healthy eating means just another fad diet; and it's all about weight loss. Achieving optimum health is altogether different. That weight loss happens is a bonus, but the goal is to learn to cooperate with all the natural systems of the body.

Create Your Plan

No lifestyle change ever happens by accident. It will require thought and purposeful planning. It will require preparation and action. Either in a notebook or on your computer, map out your plan of action. Create a start date and chart your progress for at least six weeks.

Your plan will include gradual changes in food habits, exercise, rest, and possibly finding an accountability partner. (Everyone needs encouragement.)

This plan will also include obstacles. Think them out ahead of time. What mental blocks might hinder your progress? Write these out in your planning journal, identify them, face them and push through them. Facing such obstacles will equip you to be prepared for them. (Avoid being blindsided.) Perhaps your obstacle is your dread that you might have to give up every food that you love. Or that you've tried all the diets and nothing ever works for you. Isolate the negative thinking and put them to rest once and for all.

Start in the Kitchen

Did you know your kitchen has been usurped by the food industry? It's time to get aggressive and take it back. This is an important room in your home. Treat it with respect. Start by slowly eliminating the fake foods, the empty calories, and the poisons that now fill your cupboards and pantry.

Look at the labels. Do you see *life* there? Or a long list of chemicals? Do you want your foods prepared in your kitchen or in some far-off food manufacturer's laboratory? Learn how to exchange healthy foods for the dead ones. One well-known nutritionist/physician says, "If it was grown on a plant, not made in a plant, you can keep it in your kitchen." This is excellent advice. The key is to stay away from food-like substances that have no nutrition.

We've been duped into thinking that it's faster and easier to create dinner out of a box or package, than making it from scratch. Time to change that thinking. There are myriads of highly-nutritious meals that can be put together in a few minutes. The main requirement is a change in mindset. When you make a meal from scratch, you know exactly what is in it. Not true with pre-packaged meals.

Be on the watch for dangerous foods such as high-fructose corn syrup, bleached white flour, refined white sugar, artificial sweeteners, and any hydrogenated fats and oils.

In the Grocery Aisles

Change your kitchen, then change your shopping habits. Our grocery stores have become virtual nutritional wastelands. Shop the perimeters of the store. You are now on a survival mission; search for life. Fill your cart with living foods and foods that are fresh, such as raw or frozen fruits and vegetables, fresh fish and meats. Avoid the processed foods that have no life – no nutritional value.

Curb the Caffeine

Because coffee is socially acceptable, few people understand how caffeine upsets the systems in the body. Many deeper health problems (such as underlying stress) can be masked and hidden by using coffee as a picker-upper. Just as the caffeine give a boost, it then causes an even worse *downer*. This works to confuse the nervous system. The majority of people who are addicted to caffeine have poor sleep cycles. Natural sleep is the best sleep.

One way to know whether or not you are addicted is if you experience distinct withdrawals when you have not had your caffeine fix. This is a definite sign. If this describes you, be sure to include caffeine reduction in your plan to move toward optimum health.

Exercise

As was mentioned in the previous chapter, exercise will be a close second to changes in eating habits in your journey to heart-health. Find an activity that is fun for you. It might be biking, tennis, swimming, racquet ball, working out at the gym, or simply taking a brisk walk. If it's enjoyable to you, there's more of a chance that you'll stick with it.

Many people, who for years have been adverse to regular exercise, are surprised at the differences they experience after adopting their own exercise routine. Their mood is elevated, their thinking is clearer, their creativity is heightened, their energy levels are greater, their sleep is peaceful and natural, and many of their food cravings (for junk foods) are curbed. But best of all, there's a feeling of empowerment – of being in control.

Find Your Support Group

If you are spending most of your time with people who are overweight, inactive, and unproductive, this is probably not the best group to be on your accountability team. You must find at least one or two like-minded individuals with whom you can interact. This is so you can cheer one another on. When you don't feel like getting up off the couch on a dark winter evening, it will take a like-minded friend to show up at your door ready to encourage you to go to the gym together.

Trying to go it alone can be setting yourself up for failure. Unless you are an extremely motivated self-starter, you will be more assured of success by having a support group. Especially in the early days. Later on, when you are at the top of your game, you'll need to no encouragement to go exercise – you can't wait to get there!

As you can see, there are many ways within your power to control cholesterol, and most of them are quite easy and inexpensive. They are certainly less expensive than over-the-counter drugs or prescriptions. And have no side effects – other than increased health and a sense of well being.

Conclusion

In our culture, we know more about how to care for a car than how to care for our bodies. We wouldn't treat our vehicles with as much disregard as we do our bodies. Much of the knowledge of past generations of what is required to be whole and healthy has been lost in the myriads of hyped up ads and brightly packaged processed foods.

What has been presented in this book could be considered primary prevention. Prevention is a much wiser step than relying on a pill to fix our health problems.

You have only one body and only one heart. Heart transplants are extremely expensive not to mention highly risky. So the best plan is to take excellent care of the one and only heart that was given to you.

Whether or not you are convinced that cholesterol is wholly good or wholly bad becomes somewhat irrelevant when you simply focus on adopting a healthy lifestyle.
It's time for you to take control.

Here's to your optimum health.

To work with Michael Von Irvin or make comments contact
help@writersprofitguide.com

9 781794 450899